# Stuttering

## *The Nature and a Practical Approach to the Treatment*

## A. N. Okonoboh

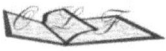

Olefaniel Publishers

**ALSO BY A. N. OKONOBOH**

*The Homecoming*
*Daggers in a Teacup*
*Words of Wisdom*

# Suttering

*The Nature and a Practical Approach to the Treatment*

**Olefaniel Publishers,**
an imprint of Olefaniel Ventures,
1 Osumba Street, by Church Bus Stop,
Igando, Lagos, 100001, Nigeria.

Tel: **+2348036846285**
aihebholooria@yahoo.com


ISBN: 9781521026373

To

Them. The speak volumes without words

Thanks to:

Ferdinand Inyang Otu, Sehinde Ilegbusi, Faith Okonoboh, Femi Fakorede, Endurance Okonoboh and Dr. Pius E. Akhimien

# Contents.

# BREATH CONTROL

BREATHING plays a very important role in human speech. The speech organs and the participatory muscles in the respiratory system gradually release the air of our breath. The system is so efficient that there is usually no need to breathe in more rapidly to sustain our speech. This however is not to oversimplify the task of speaking. A lot of complex activities go on in our bodies unknown to us. They are natural and not burdensome. Yet the quality of speech is sometimes determined by the ability to control the breath. Conscious control of the breath is even more vital especially when there is a speech challenge or impediment. Some of these speech challenges are stammer, lisping, consonant issues, etc. In this program, we will be focusing mainly on stammer and how to stop it.

What is stammer? In the context of this course, stammer is the inability to coordinate the speech organs to say the first sound. This usually results in stopping and attempting to say the word several times before saying it correctly.

Stammer however, does not refer to any distortion of the organs of speech themselves.

These organs in most cases are in good working order. That is why it is no wonder that a stutterer may speak fluently on certain occasions, but dysfluently at others.

There is a gene for stammer recently discovered by some scientists around the year 2012. This means that stammer can be a family trait. But even in many families where some children show the trait, hardworking parents have been able to help such children to resolve the problem in them. This goes to show that even though stammer could be present in the gene, the environment to a large extent, level of anxiety and stress determine whether a person shows it or lives with the trait or not. Knowing what to do, consciously doing them, or having someone reminding us to do them are all actions that work against the stammer genetic traits.

Stuttering is also associated with about three other causes. Neurological abnormalities, trauma and phobias and anxieties are in the number.

Learning to control the breath is where it starts. As already mentioned, breathing affects our performance in speeches. This could be seen in the depth and the clarity of voice, speech pace, sound pitch as well as the stability of the voice. For example, a shallow breathing causes a clipped or high-pitched sound, while a deep breath produces a thunderous one.

Many people are not concerned about controlling their breath. It is usually because they speak normally and the mechanisms for their speeches are driven by nature. But if you are a stammerer, you have good reasons to care. To learn to speak smoothly, you need to consciously control your breath until your speech becomes normalised. This lesson will show you just what breath control is all about and what you should do to gain the skill.

FILLING THE LUNGS: There are two kinds of breathing. They are: 1. Breathing from the chest and 2. Breathing from the lungs. Either of the two kinds affects the speech negatively or positively.

When a person breathes from the chest, he fills only the upper part of the lungs. This affects the amount of air he has in him to speak and in turn the quality of the sound produced. Breathing is often this way when a person is anxious. Then the muscles become taut including those for speech. This situation is responsible for a high rate of word jam in a stutter.

To breath from the lungs on the other hand, the lower part of the lungs is filled first. Then the rising of the rib cage is observed as the filling of the upper part followed. Breathing from the lungs neutralises the tension in the muscles. And it is recommended for a stutter. It also increases confidence and poise.

Having come to understand the kinds of breathings there are, what can you say about your regular breathing at present? You can start now to breath from the lungs if you have observed differently. Fill the lower part of your lungs. Then, your ribs will expand to fill the upper part as you continue to suck in air. Consciously avoid filling only the upper part of your lungs.

VERIFY YOUR BREATHING: To find out where breathing originates, place a palm of your hand on the lower part of your belly. It should rise and you will feel pressure at the waistline before you observe the rib cage expanding to fill the upper part of your lungs.

Breath control is the primary level of this program. It helps to relax the muscles of the throat, the jaws, the vocal cord and those of the rest of the body. It brings a person to the right mind frame too. Such calmness is groundwork for the muscles around the vocal cord or pharynx to adjust freely. This leads to fewer cases of word jam and less struggle to make the first sound.

Probably you have started already, to practice breathing properly from the lungs. Why not stand before a mirror and start discussing a subject that often poses some challenge. Does the mirror say that your neck is still taut and stiff? What about your shoulders? Of course, your breathing deep will eventually correct the situation.

Another indication of poise and calmness is the use of body members such as the hands, the legs, the eyelids, etc, when talking. If they move involuntarily, awkwardly, then pay more attention to your breathing.

Practice! Practice! Practice! Controlling the breath is not going to be automatic. But with practice and conscious efforts, you will surely gain it and the ability to coordinate your speech organs. And you will acqire the ability to speak fluently.

1. Every day for three months, place a palm of your hand on the lower part of your abdomen for several minutes. Practice filling your lungs until you feel pressure in the lower

part of your abdomen as it rises. Do this also while speaking.

2. At different times of the day for three months, practice relaxing the following muscles: a) Throat muscles, b) The jaws muscles, and c) The shoulders muscles. Do this also while speaking.

# THE ART OF SPEAKING.

STAMMER is not a lack of knowledge of language structure. The stutter understands that spoken languages are made up of words. A word may have one or more syllable. And syllables are smaller units of words that produce their own sounds independently. (Examples: Perception = Per-cep-tion and Independently = In-de-pen-dent-ly) A stammerer's problem is failure to assign a distinct sound to each of these smaller units in their speeches. Therefore, the help he needs is about how to handle words and their components in a speech.

*CHANGING PERCEPTION*

A stutterer is often not patient enough to give consideration to the important roles the sounds of syllables play in a speech. They speak very fast when it flows or swallow some sounds when there is an obstacle. Speaking in this manner, violates the proper use of words units in the speech art. For example, when a person speaks too fast, words are run together which is called slurring. The sounds of many syllables are either omitted or confused as a consequence. This makes it very likely to hit an obstacle on the way. Similarly, when some sounds are swallowed, which is often termed muffle, sounds of syllables are also lost in the process. Most of the time, this leads to the self-interruptions that a stutter experiences. It is strongly recommended that a stutter work hard to change his perception and give syllables their proper functions when speaking.

### DIFFERING SPEECH SCHEMES

Why does a stutterer speak rapidly or muffles sounds? He has two types of speeck blueprints stored in his brain. They are the fluency schedule and the stammer scheme. When he speaks fast, his brain has picked up the the fluency schedule. And when he is jerky and muffling, the brain is utilizing the stammer scheme. This is a choice that is determined by the environment, emotional status or the physical frailty.

## ADJUSTING TO THE RULES

Adjusting actually takes patience and efforts. But the result is clearly seen at every level. It doesn't hide. The more the effort that is put into making progress the clearer the advancement that will be seen.

**1. LEARN PATIENCE.** Suppress the urge to begin speaking immediately to satisfy a listener (one person or an audience of more people) when there is need to respond or say something. This is not easy because it is likely what you have been doing all your life. But it is highly recommended. Start learning not to rush yourself for whatever reason. Let the reason wait. Instead, before beginning to talk, take a moment to inhale deeply several times. This relaxes your muscles as already discussed in the proceeding lesson. Then start slowly and continue at a very slow and comfortable pace.

**2. COUNTING ALL THE SOUNDS.** Following the examples given at the opening paragraph, mentally break the words of your speech into syllables. Then allow the sound of each of the syllables to come out distinctly in your speech. You might be frightened by the result, a terrible lack of flow. It may even appear that you are learning allover again to speak like a small child. Do not be discouraged or feel shamed. It is rather evidence that you are making progress. In time, you will resume a normal flow of speech and without the words jam that used to make you stammer. It is as effective as reinstalling a program on the computer.

Unlike some shocking vision or experiences that provoke chemical brain imprint, the skills discussed so far are not automatically picked up by the brain. So, effort and practice are very vital to replace the habits of slurring and muffling. They will also help you to be more patient. And if you can learn to count all the sound of a word no matter the affectation, your jaws and tongue will adjust to normal movement. Each day, you will see your victory over stammer very close.

When you stumble what will you do? This will be treated in the succeeding lesson.

### Exercises

1. Look for opportunity everyday for three months, to converse with someone. Observe how slow and patient you are each time you

have opportunity to speak. Then score yourself with your performance over a hundred.

2. Let someone listen while you speak. Have him check for evidence of slurring, muffling and the degree of syllabic sound clarity. Let them score you with your performance over a hundred.

3. Reduce the following words to their syllables

Community. ........ ..... ..... ...... ..... .... ..... ..... .... ....

Broadcasting ....... .......... ......... ............... ......... ... ...

Comprehensively ..................... ............................ ....

Organization. ....... ........... ........... ........ ............. ......

Idiosyncrasy. ......... ........ ......... ......... ...... .... ....
... ............ ...............

4. Make your own note of words you wish to break down to their component syllables. (Use worksheet below) Practice sounding each syllable distinctly. Continue to do this until you are through with this program

# DEALING WITH COMMON OBSTACLES.

THIS lesson is designed to help you identify the major obstacles that impede the flow of speech and the practical action to take under each situation. It is in three levels: 1. An extemporaneous discussion, 2. Interruption handling skills and 3. A second extemporaneous discusion. The benefits of recording midgets will also be introduced at this time. It will concluded with your bearing as a speaker.

*AN EXTEMPORANEOUS DISCUSSION.*

**SELECTING YOUR MATERIALS**: Select a topic from a book that deals with one of your favourite subjects. Take a day or two to study the selected topic until you are familiar with the main ideas. Next, make a note. The note should not be detailed. It should contain only a few words and phrases that at a glance may help you remember the main ideas in the the topic you have studied though not in the exact wordings of the author.

**PREPARING YOUR MATERIAL:** Practice your delivery out aloud in front of a mirror using the small note in your hand. Try to apply the skills you already learned. Take several deep breaths. Observe that the muscles of your shoulders, the neck and the jaws are relaxed enough. Observe your level of patience. Start slowly and make sure the sound of every syllable come out precisely. Remember not to care about the lack of flow. Fluency will return later by itself. Take ten to thirty minutes each day to prepare your delivery out aloud, until you are personally moved by the material.

SELECTING YOUR AUDIENCE: Decide who you will like to discuss your material with. At first, it is usually best to look for a friendly audience. Think of one or two friendly faces among your friends and arrange to present your speech to them through extemporaneous delivery style. The audience number might be increased in time as desired. They will also come from any circle later. By then you will have gained confidence and poise.

THE SPEECH PRESENTATION: Stand upright before your seated audience. Take a moment and take a few deep breaths. Look at your audience and pick out the most friendly of the faces. Start slowly, speaking to that one first, until you are absorbed into your speech.

## *INTERRUPTION HANDLING SKILLS*

(Have you completed the first assignment on extemporaneous discourse? Note: If you have not, please do not proceed to reading the next section below. You must identify core problems inhibiting normal speech flow first. Then you will be guided on how to resolve them.)

Did you notice something about your final delivery in front of your friend(s)? No doubt, you have recorded marked improvement in your speech. You were more relaxed because your muscles were calmer than you ever experienced. You avoided rushing yourself too, because you tried to be patient and was speaking slowly. And your words were also not slurred nor were sounds of syllables muffled. This is well commendable.

We observed something else. You know it too but not in the terms that we do because you cannot explain it. It seems always to be in the verge of escaping you. They are the major obstacles largely responsible for a stammerer's jerky speech. They come to play each time they stumble over words.

1. Inability to pause at once

2. Regression

3. Semantic noise

If your stammer situation is the serious type, you had interruptive word jam several times during your speech delivery assignment above. What did you do? You went back in the sentence struggling to repeat some of what you already said. This is called regression. Also, you did not pause for a breath. There were crasks at words, instead. In some cases, some sounds were employed to fill some long empty pauses. Some examples of such sounds are "em," "you know," "so," "uh," "you see," etc. These unwanted sounds are called semantic noise.

What is the proper thing to do whenever stammer interrupts your statement?

1. PAUSE IMMEDIATELY. Take a quick and deep breath. Then start to speak again, at a slow and relaxed pace.

2. AVOID REGRESSION. There is no need to go back and repeat some words or phrases when you resume your speech. Begin with exactly the last word where the interruption occurred.

3. COMPLETELY ELIMINATE SEMANTIC NOISE. You already know what those noise are, any unwanted sound intended to fill a long and embarrassing pause–"em," "you know," "so,"

"uh," "you see," etc. They do not contribute anything to the objective of your speech. They rather distort it and make them awkward. So, no matter how long a pause, it is best to leave the interval blank. You can verify the truthfulness of this matter by making a recording of both situations.

SUMMARY NOTE: 1. Immediate pause, 2. Avoid regression, and 3. Eliminate semantic noise.

*A SECOND EXTEMPORANEOUS DISCUSSION*

At this point, take another speech assignment.

Follow the same method as in the first assignment to select a different topic, gather and prepare the materials, and the rest of them. In your delivery in front of your audience, show that you have applied the foregoing skills on handling interruptions during your days of preparations.

## Make your comments

Pausing immediately ............ .......... .......... .............. ..
.......................................................................
.......................................................................
.......................................................................
.......................................................................
.......................................................................
.......................................................................

Level of regression ............ ........, .....,...,. ............ ......
.......................................................................
.......................................................................
.......................................................................
.......................................................................
.......................................................................
.......................................................................

Elimination of semantic noise ........ ....... ..........
.......................................................................
.......................................................................
.......................................................................
.......................................................................
.......................................................................
.......................................................................

## BENEFITS OF RECORDING MIDGETS

Recording and preserving your voice is very important in this course. It helps to keep track of your progress. This is not to say that it is impossible to monitor your progress without recordings. No. You can daily see the positive changes in your speech.

Recordings will however give you a more graphic view of these improvements. With it, you can make comparisons. Areas of serious flaws would easily be brought to your notice. And newer recordings will give you much encouragement.

We are fortunate today to be living at a time when recording midgets and devices are there for the taking. Why, even the simplest of mobile phones has an audio recorder built into it. So, getting a device won't be a challenge. Put these to good advantage.

## YOUR BEARING AS A SPEAKER

The body members should be consciously controlled. It is very awkward to shuffle the feet and look at the floor while talking to someone. It is not a pleasant sight to stick out the tongue or slap the thighs or the shoulders of a listener standing nearby. It is also not a good posture to shuffle the hand in and out of the pocke or to allow the eyes to bulge while speaking. But one or more of these happen frequently, especially to a stutter. They show nervousness and a lack of poise.

Remember though that you want to impart something valuable to your listener. But if your bearing is awkward when you speak, the attention of your listener will shift from what you are saying. Instead, he will focus on you and start to sympathize. And for you, this is not going to be pleasant. You may look stupid to yourself and become dejected.

That is why you need to care very much about your bearing when you speak. The only ways to solve this problem is being alert to what you do with your body members and using your breaths to calm your nerves.

Be assured that with time, the frequency of word jams requiring pauses will diminish. Noise will be completely eliminated. The gap of pauses between statements will close. Also, make generous recordings of your voice from time to time. Use them to monitor your progress. Preserve them for future references.

**Stammer**

Work very hard to manage your bearing. And gradually, fluency will return to your speech.

# HOW OTHERS CAN HELP

*A friend.*

IS there someone with whom you spend a considerable amount of time every day? Is the person one interested in seeing you succeed in this battle one day? And would he be willing to be of some assistance? If yes is your answer to all three questions, you are in good company.

Assign him a role. He can always give you a signal to pause each time you are trying to force yourself to continue an obstructed statement. This will complement your own effort to remember to take some appropriate actions. Being conscious of what you are doing at any time is very important.

My speech ratings today

_____

_____

_____

_____

_____

_____

_____

_____

_____

_____

## The Role of Parents

"One begins to coil the tail of a dog when it is still a puppy," says an *Ishan* proverb. So, when your little child gives evidence of stammer, get at work on time at that tender age. And help him from infancy to break the unkind yoke of stammer.

Researchers have established that the root of almost all cases of stammer goes back to childhood. Therefore, if parents are keen at playing their roles early enough in the child's life, cases of stutter today would be reduced drastically.

With the flexible mind of a child, it is not a difficult thing to correct this defect in him. All that needs to be done is reminding him to pause when he cracks at a word, and then encouraging him to say it again. You may also wish to help him with the statement at hand by saying it yourself, after which you encourage him to say it after you. In this way, developing the ability to speak fluently would not be a problem for the child as he grows. The parents that have come to us have all recorded success in this regard.

Never make the mistake of leaving the matter of stammer in your child to chance. Do not put your hope in the belief that he will give it up as he grows. Granted, stammer is short-lived in most children. Still, you can never tell which child will carry it further. It is as difficult as trying to identify the cock among unhatched eggs.

Do your best therefore, to forestall problem for your child. And you will never regret the efforts you invested.

# CONSONANT ERRORS

CONSONANT error is the loss of certain consonants or the misreading of one as another in the sound of a word according to the degree of tongue rolling ability. The problem is mostly hereditary.

For a number of reasons, the problem is not an alarming one. In some cases, certain ethnics or languages do not have some consonants because of the language structure. And anybody raised in these languages inherits this loss. So it won't bother many natives except a few who make effort to regain the loss. The Yoruba speaking tribe of Nigeria is a good example. The Yoruba language structure does not have room for the letter "V." So whenever a situation calls for "V" the Yorubas improvise "F."

But for a person who must speak languages other than his native tongue, there are compelling reasons for concern. It is not just enough to speak another language but the way it is spoken matters a lot. Improper enunciation of words can result in broken ideas or even a change of meaning altogether.

Can the word "Glory" retain its distinctive sound if it is pronounced by someone without "L" and "R" sound? What is likely to be heard is "Goi," which can easily be mistaken for "going."

How can improvement be made? Well, if you know of an Obsessive Compulsive Disorder sufferer what would you recommend for him? Stain himself with what is most repulsive to him. In a similar vein, a person who suffers from consonant errors should pick out the ones that pose challenge to him. After that is done, he should endeavour to play with each, practicing rolling the tongue to get the particular consonant sound right.

A person with "R" error can begin with ri-ri-ri... Then, rrrrrrrr... For a person who lisp, it suffices to be alert when about to pronounce "S" and "Z" and to get more room for the tongue before pronouncing them.

With dedication and practice, a person with these errors can learn to adjust and roll the tongue properly.

### Exercises

1. Several times every day, for three months practice rolling your tongue in every way. During this period, try also to sound the letters that give you special challenge.

2. Try to roll your tongue towards the sounds of certain consonants.

3. On the sheet below, list all the consonants on which you need work.

......................................................................

......................................................................

......................................................................

......................................................................

......................................................................

......................................................................

......................................................................

......................................................................

......................................................................

......................................................................

......................................................................

......................................................................

......................................................................

......................................................................

# AUTHOR'S NOTE

WE have set you on the road to the world of fluency. We have garlanded you with practical skills to deal effectively with stammer. And your quiver is filled with the right arrows. Now, we are leaving you here to become your master. So go and conquer in the midst of your enemies. Before then, let us tell you goodbye our way. We hope to hear from you again, when you will have gained the victory, when you will have been free to talk as you like it and when you will look for us to tell 'Thank you.'

Farewell!